BATTLING BREAST CANCER
WITH
NUTRITION

Heather Gabbert, MS, RD, LD, CD
Kathy Beach, RN
Christopher M. Lee, MD

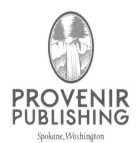

PROVENIR
PUBLISHING
Spokane, Washington

www.provenirpublishing.com

Battling Breast Cancer with Nutrition

Copyright © 2013 by Provenir Publishing, LLC
Printed in the United States of America

This book includes text adapted from books in the Living and Thriving with... series published by Provenir Publishing with the editor's permission.

Published by Provenir Publishing, LLC, P. O. Box 211, Greenacres, WA 99016-0211

Production Credits

Lead Editor: Christopher Lee

Production Director: Amy Harman

Art Director and Illustration: Micah Harman

Cover Design: Micah Harman

Printing History: April 2013, First Edition.

This book is dedicated to our patients and their families,
who inspire us every day in their cancer fight.

Contents

It is nearly impossible to find someone who doesn't have a family member or close friend affected by breast cancer. Worldwide, breast cancer accounts for approximately 23% of all cancers in women. Breast cancer is more than 100 times more common in women than in men, although men tend to have poorer outcomes due to delays in diagnosis.

The general prognosis and survival rates for women with breast cancer vary greatly depending on the cancer type, stage, treatment, and geographical location of the patient. Survival rates in the Western world are high because of modern treatments and access to care. In developing countries, however, survival rates are much poorer.

It is very common for patients with a cancer diagnosis to have many questions about nutrition and diet. In fact, this is one of the main ways that you (or your loved one) can aid yourself in the battle with cancer. The cancer can inhibit your body's ability to heal, decrease your energy, and decrease your immune system. By optimizing diet and nutrition, research has shown that outcomes of surgery, radiation, and chemotherapy are improved. This leads to improved cure rates, better cancer treatment outcomes, and greater ability for the body to heal and rebound from the effects of cancer therapy.

The goal of this text is to empower patients during their fight with cancer. By studying these practical approaches to health and nutrition, you can aid your cancer treatment team in your therapies. This is not meant to be a substitute for standard modern cancer treatments, but the goal is to provide you with further tools to fight cancer and improve your ability to heal from the cancer and the cancer treatments. Of course, this tool should be used in the context of your other treatments and we recommend that each patient discuss their individual health needs and objectives with their care providers.

Chapter One

Focusing On Nutrition

Breast cancer. Two words that can rock your world. "You have breast cancer." Four words that can cause your life to flash before your eyes. It's unsettling to say the least. It is interesting that many patients come in feeling desperate and at a loss, but it is those same patients that

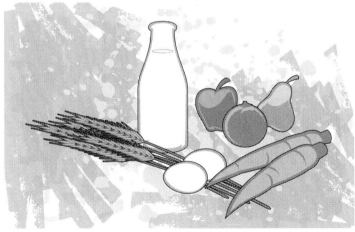

Focusing on nutrition can be the best thing that you can do for yourself during cancer therapy.

grab cancer by the tail and say, "Hey, I'm not going to let cancer bully me. It's time to fight and I am going to do what I can to beat you or at the very least, control you so I can live my life!" Following some nutritional and lifestyle recommendations can help in fighting breast cancer. Some things that can help make you feel a little more in control of what may feel like an out of control situation are laid out on the following pages. What you chose to eat can have a strong impact on fighting this cancer. Your immune system is what fights off illnesses and disease. By making the best choices nutritionally, you can maximize your immune system's fighting potential, making you the best cancer fighter you can be. It's all about boosting your immune system, fighting inflammation and decreasing challenges to your immune system so it can focus on the current battle at hand.

Knowledge is power. It's time to empower you with knowledge in this fight against cancer. Arm yourself with knowledge. Let's get to it!

American Institute Of Cancer Research (AICR) Findings-Breast Cancer

Visit *AICR.org* or *foodandcancerreport.org* to download, for free, the findings from the 2007, 2nd Expert Report. The information provided by the AICR expert report was broken down into two sections for breast cancer. The evidence and judgments were divided into "pre-menopause" and "post-menopause."

There is convincing evidence that lactation decreases risk of breast cancer, and intake of alcoholic drinks increases regardless if one is either pre or post-menopause. There is probable evidence that body fatness decreases risk during pre-menopausal period, while body fatness, post-menopause, increases risk of breast cancer. The reason being the body fat distribution that occurs with menopause is mainly in the abdominal area. There is apparently more visceral fat (inside the abdominal cavity) which harbors those toxins and harmful substances. It is also known that a waistline of >35 inches for females is a risk factor for cancers, heart disease and other diseases. Physical activity/exercise decrease risk of breast cancer both pre and post-menopause.

What are you supposed to do with this information? Well, basically, this means to eat more foods that are anti-inflammatory, immune boosting, lower in fat, and mostly plant based, and drink less or no alcohol. Physical activity is a must as well. Specific foods are found to be more anti-inflammatory than others, which is why a variety of nutritional intake is recommended. A couple of powerful nutrients are selenium and quercitin, which are referred to as flavonoids, or more specifically flavonols. Selenium is found more in certain nuts and seeds and fish, while flavonols are found in vegetables and darker colored fruits. Both selenium and quercitin are naturally occurring antioxidants and are anti-inflammatory. Please see below for lists of foods containing these flavonoids. Intake of these foods are encouraged, but please talk to your doctor, naturopathic doctor, or dietitian about taking quercitin supplementation.

As for the physical activity recommendations, get moving more! Be more active and get that blood pumping! Physical activity helps directly and indirectly to decrease cancer risk. Also, it can improve mental state or mood, release negative energy and help fight inflammation. The federal guidelines for exercise are great and relatively easy to attain. It is recommended we get physically active at least 150 minutes a week or do 75 minutes a week of vigorous exercise each week. In addition to that, you should do weight training (just about 15 minutes) twice

Nurse's Note:

Always consult your doctor before starting a new exercise program.

3

a week. See!? You can do this! It may not be so easy if you are undergoing treatment and are fatigued, however, try to be as active as possible to help maintain muscle mass. Monitor your fatigue level and just do what you can. The resistance bands are great for helping you to keep muscle tone and can be done while sitting in the comforts of your own home. You must be careful if you have recently undergone surgery for breast or tumor removal, and please note if you have any signs of lymphedema you should talk to a physical therapist specialized in this area about the amount of movement that is allowed, to safely avoid making lymphedema any worse.

Alcohol intake should be limited, or none at all. WHAT?!! "What about that glass of wine every night I have while making dinner?!", you ask. Well, that should be OK. For females, one, 6 ounce glass of wine is considered "in moderation." Some of you right now are screaming, "More like a drop!" But when looking at the information there is convincing evidence to support such recommendations. Sincerely think about decreasing intake of wine and other alcoholic beverages.

Another recommendation is to decrease body fatness by decreasing the amount of inflammatory fats consumed and increasing that physical activity level. Read on and more detailed information on kinds of fats to consume and more powerful information on immune boosting nutrition is ahead.

Selenium Containing Foods:

- Brazil nuts
- Sunflower seeds
- Tuna (canned light tuna in oil)
- Cod (cooked)

Quercitin Containing Foods:

- Apples
- Red or black grapes
- Blueberries
- Blackberries
- Cherries
- Onions (raw yields 30% more quercitin than cooked)
- Scallions
- Kale
- Broccoli
- Green tea and red wine from dark grapes (as stated by Linus Pauling Institute)

    Go to livestrong.com for more information on quercitin if you like.

Chapter Two

Immune Boosting Nutrition

Make every bite count. Well, almost every bite. Follow the 80/20 rule. Eighty percent of the time you should make every bite count. Make the best choice for what you decide to fuel your body with. So often we are on the go, or in a hurry, and making unconscious decisions regarding our nutritional intake. Think about it. Is what you are eating doing anything for your body and your fight against cancer? If not, maybe you should think about making some changes in your food selections. That's not to say you can't enjoy those foods that, let's be honest, aren't good for you but they sure taste good and make you feel happy. You can. These are the foods that you have only around 20% of the time. Enjoying birthday celebrations, dessert out with girlfriends, or any number of social occasions, will most likely involve chips, dips and drink choices that you seldom consume. It's OK to enjoy these moments. Make a conscious effort to eat the best you can most of the time, so you can enjoy these special moments and the "not so good" nutrition choices that accompany these occasions without the guilt. It's all part of a healthy eating experience. It's all part of life, as is this current fight you've got on your hands.

Mainly, regarding your diet, the focus should lie on getting back to the basics. Having less processed foods is where it's at! When buying boxed/convenience foods, select those with less ingredients. Take ice cream for example. It can be a source of protein and calcium, but has high content of fat, therefore, only consume it occasionally. What you should look at, though, is how many ingredients went into making it. Buy the ice cream containing only five ingredients or so. Breyers All Natural is a good example of this. I'm not saying it's okay to eat ice cream all the time, but it is okay sometimes, especially if there are no chemicals/preservatives added to it. This is just an example. In general, focus on eating whole grains, dark and brightly colored fruits and vegetables, plant proteins, lean animal protein sources, fish (especially those high in Omega 3 fatty acids), and other good fats which are listed below. The idea is to balance out carbs and protein at each meal, mini meal or snack. Also by incorporating the good fats into your diet, this will help in sparing the protein you take in for healing and repair.

Whole Grains:

When choosing whole grain foods, select those that have been the least processed or are closer to their natural state. Some examples of whole grains include: brown rice, wild rice, whole wheat pasta, quinoa, quinoa pasta, high fiber cereals (hot or cold) containing 5 grams or more fiber per serving, and breads made from whole grain flour, having 3 grams of fiber or more per slice. Whole grain flour being the first ingredient listed. Whole grains have complex carbohydrates in them which are needed by our bodies for energy. They also have protein in them. Quinoa, for example, has 6-10 grams of protein per ½ cup. Give it a try if you haven't already.

Produce:

It is recommended that 5 or more servings of fruit and vegetables be consumed each day. This is challenging for a lot of people. A recommendation that is easy to adhere to is to add a fruit or vegetable to every meal, mini meal or snack eaten during the day. Try to eat small meals, every 3 hours or so. At each of these add a serving of produce. Aim for 5 servings a day of dark or brightly colored produce.

Some of the best choices include:

- Broccoli, cauliflower, brussels sprouts, kale and bok choy. These are called cruciferous vegetables and they contain isothiocyanates, specifically Indole-3-Carbinol. This is a cancer fighting compound and should be consumed on a daily basis!

- Berries of all varieties.

- Carrots and orange colored produce for the carotenoids. (Carotenoid-containing foods are especially good for fighting lung cancer!)

- Red grapes for the resveratrol.

This is a short list of some of the most powerful cancer fighting produce available at grocery stores. It is highly recommended you have your own garden if you can, and grow produce organically. Another thing that should always be mentioned when discussing produce is to wash it in a vinegar and water solution. Wash produce using a solution of 1 Tablespoon vinegar (any kind) in 4 cups of water. This will help to pull off 95-99% of the cancer-causing pesticides used in the farming of the produce. For the thin skinned fruits and hard to wash vegetables, it is better to go organic because it is difficult to completely clean these off. This decreases challenges to your immune system, one less thing to worry about.

Plant Proteins:

Foods of plant origin are high in fiber, vitamins, minerals, antioxidants, beneficial plant compounds, and prebiotic fibers to help support healthy intestinal bacteria balance. Plant based foods are the basis for an anti-inflammatory diet. Beans, legumes, lentils, nuts, seeds, soy foods—these are all sources of protein coming from a plant source. GO FOR IT! Add these to your salads, soups, chili's, or make a bean burger, etc.

Animal Proteins:

Nurse's Note:

Ask your doctor or nurse about nutrition supplements.

Protein from animal sources is allowed also, but be sure to buy leaner cuts of meat, chicken and other poultry with no skin, and go organic when it comes to purchasing red meat and dairy products containing fat. Buy grass fed cattle because it is higher in Omega-3 fatty acids which are anti-inflammatory. Animal foods, in general, contain higher amount of Omega-6 fatty acids which are pro-inflammatory so the goal is to decrease intake of animal based foods, and increase intake of plant based foods and fish, especially those high in Omega-3 fats (sources listed below). Why avoid processed/cured meats? They contain nitrates/nitrite which are known to cause cancer. This cancer causing agent is used in hams, deli meats, hot dogs, bacon and sausages. Select nitrate-free products such as Hormel Natural Selections deli meat, bacon, etc and limit intake. It can be found in the deli meat section of the grocery store.

List Of Protein Foods:

Beans, legumes, lentils – Typical serving size is ¼ cup which equals 7 grams protein. Increase bean intake – try hummus spread, made from garbanzo beans (aka chickpeas).

Nuts, seeds – ¼ cup = 7 grams protein. If nuts and seeds are not tolerated, grind nuts into a spread at your local grocery store. The nut grinders are usually found in the "Health Food" section of the grocery stores by the "All Natural" items.

Soy foods are considered safe for all breast cancer patients to a certain degree. One to three servings of soy foods are allowed for breast cancer patients who are estrogen receptor positive (ER+). What is not recommended are the concentrated forms of soy, such as soy protein powders and soy protein isolates found in many energy bars and meal replacement drinks. Some examples of serving sizes of soy foods include: 1 cup soy milk, 4 ounces tofu, 1/3 cup soy nuts,

6 ounces soy yogurt, ½ cup textured vegetable protein and 1 cup edamame (in pod). It would be okay to have 1-3 servings/day of these soy foods.

Milks and spreads/nut butter made from plant foods – Almond milk, soy milk, soy yogurt, or may grind any nut to make a nut butter at your local grocery store. (Please note as stated previously, intake of soy foods considered safe at 1-3 servings/day if cancer if hormone based; estrogenic (ER/PR+). A serving size of a nut butter is typically 2 tablespoons.

Fish, especially wild caught salmon, tuna, halibut, mackerel and rainbow trout, for their Omega-3 fatty acid content. Omega-3s, as stated previously, are a natural anti-inflammatory and should be consumed 2-3 times per week. Other fish do not contain high levels of Omega-3s, however, are lean protein sources, 4 ounces being a serving of fish it provides 28 grams of protein. High mercury levels have been found in marine sources, so it is suggested to eat fish only 2-3 times per week. Omega-3 supplementation is recommended for this reason.

Eggs are a high quality protein. Each egg has about 5-7 grams of protein. Suggest having 5 eggs a week and unlimited egg whites.

Chicken and turkey – no skin, are lean protein sources. Each ounce has 7 grams protein.

LEAN cuts of red meat – Sirloin, ground sirloin for burgers vs ground chuck, and flank steak for fajitas, for example, would be okay for consumption. Also, look for grass-fed cattle as this meat will have more Omega-3s vs the inflammatory Omega-6s. The AICR generally recommends limiting intake of red meat, to about 3 servings per week.

Greek yogurt has about 12-14 grams protein in it and four to five different strains of live cultures (probiotics) which will help to normalize gut flora and promote bacteria balance in the intestines.

Low or no-fat dairy – Skim milk, 1% milk, low fat, skim mozzarella, etc. When buying a fat-containing animal product it is recommended to go organic. Look for the following statement or something similar on the label, "No hormones or antibiotics were given to this animal or used in the making of this product." Keep in mind when buying fat-containing animal foods: hormones, and toxins given to the animal are stored in the fat of the animal. (Much like humans.) The fattier the animal food, the more likely you are to consume the bad things stored in the fat of the animal. Safer to go organic when it comes to fat-containing animal products. Wise to spend your money on organic meats and dairy products.

Good Fats:

Lowering dietary intake of Omega-6 fats (mostly animal foods) while raising intake of Omega-3 fats will help to shift the body into "anti-inflammatory" mode. What are good sources of Omega-3s? High Omega-3 foods include wild caught salmon, tuna, halibut, mack-

Nurse's Note:

Freezing your favorite foods may help you plan your meals in advance.

Nurse's Note:

Remember, because caffeine is a diuretic, it can actually dehydrate you. You may want to cut down or eliminate caffeine completely during treatment.

erel and rainbow trout. Also, foods of plant origin will have less Omega-6 fats and some Omega-3s like walnuts and flaxseed oil. Extra virgin olive oil, canola oil and coconut oil are examples of good fats as are avocados, nuts and seeds. Daily intake of a ¼ - ½ of an avocado is recommended.

Hydration

Keeping the body hydrated is so very important every day, not just during treatment for cancer. You, in general, need 13-18 ml of non-caloric, caffeine free fluids per pound of weight each day to maintain a good hydration status. Example: 150 lbs x 13 ml/lb = 1950 ml/day which is equivalent to 8 ¼ cups per day of fluid. Monitor urine frequency, color and odor. If it looks concentrated or darker in color and has an odor, you very well may be dehydrated. On the day of chemotherapy you will receive one liter of fluid with treatment to assure you are adequately hydrated and that the chemo is flushed through your kidneys appropriately. On the other days, it is all up to you to maintain your fluid intake. If you find yourself having trouble getting enough fluid in, be sure to inform your oncologist, nurse and/or dietitian to possibly get set up for IV fluids a few days a week. Hydration is that important! It is just as important as food intake. The more vocal you are with your symptoms, the better they can be managed, so inform your health care team early and often. And work on staying hydrated as best as you can! Another thing you need to work hard on is consistent food intake all day long to fuel your body for cancer fighting!

Chapter Three

Balance, Timing, And Planning

Regulate Blood Sugar And Keep The Body Fueled!

Fueling your body consistently all day long, every day, will help to maintain an even keel throughout the day and avoid peaks and valleys associated with varying sugar intake. By staying on an even keel all day you will provide needed support to your immune system so that it can work at its best potential. Blood sugar stabilization is key. Statements like, "I don't eat breakfast." Or, "My whole life I've never eaten breakfast," are often heard and now is the time for that to change. Try to consume calories, whether it's eating or drinking, within an hour of waking. You need to wake the body up and let it know that nutrition is on the way. If you're not doing this, it is very likely that your metabolism will slow down. Another very important thing to remember is that caffeine is an appetite suppressant. Countless people have said, "I just drink black coffee all morning and I'm not hungry for anything until about 4:00 in the afternoon." The reason one can go so long without having an appetite is due, in part, to the caffeine intake as it is an appetite suppressant- not signaling the hunger cue. In actuality, you are slowing down the metabolism. What you need now is a well-oiled machine and to stay revved up to support weight maintenance as well as your immune system. We are addressing weight management and immune-boosting nutrition. To continue boosting the immune system and support your cancer fighting body, eating every 3 hours is suggested, trying never to go longer than 4 hours between intake. This will help to support blood sugar stability all day long and keep you and your immune system energized. Imagine this: your body is a wood stove. You want to keep the fire burning all day long so you need logs (protein foods) and kindling (carbohydrates) every few hours. Why do this? The answer is simple. If your body doesn't have consistent source of fuel, it will think uh-oh, I don't have anything coming in, and begin to work its magic in fueling your body, slowing things down if you will and eventually pulling from energy stores in your body. You have stored energy in your muscles and when not properly nourished you may begin to breakdown muscle. A good way to gauge muscle loss is to look at your arms. Look for atrophy (shrinking muscle mass). Notice if there is any muscle or fat loss.

Of course, monitor your weight. It is okay to lose a little bit of weight but want to avoid significant weight loss. Your oncologist and care team will be following you during and after your treatment to monitor your overall health status. Significant weight loss is indicative of the inability to meet caloric needs. The registered dietitian on the team will be alerted if you should experience significant weight loss, change in nutritional status, and/ or begin to be more symptomatic. A nutrition consult would be beneficial to address and possibly prevent or minimize symptoms you may encounter and provide you with ways to manage them. Managing side effects early can help to minimize the symptoms, thus minimizing the impact they may have on your overall nutritional status. It is very important to let your physician, nurse, dietitian, or any member of the health care team know of any or all symptoms you may be experiencing.

Chapter Four

Treating the Symptoms of Cancer or Treatment

Symptoms associated with treatment for breast cancer include: constipation (from pain meds, mostly), diarrhea, decreased or no appetite, sore throat, painful swallowing, difficulty swallowing, taste changes, nausea, vomiting, and anemia. Hair loss may occur and for some breast cancer patients, this is one of the most dreaded of symptoms simply because there is a feeling of vulnerability associated with hair loss. It is commonly stated that one doesn't wish to appear sick and when they lose their hair, it may become apparent to others that something is going on. There are many resources and people to contact regarding use of wigs, accessories and other boutique items. Be sure to talk with the social worker/

case manager or patient navigator to get familiar with all that is available to you in your community.

Esophagitis may occur if radiation is part of the treatment and the location of the tumor is near the esophagus. Oftentimes, radiation therapy will be used to shrink the tumor and if the tumor is located near the esophagus, it may cause painful swelling of the esophageal area. Esophagitis is inflammation of the esophagus and can make it painful or difficult in getting foods all the way down. During radiation the body will naturally send lubrication to the site of radiation, as well as send inflammation to this site in attempts to heal. Sure the body is trying to heal this area, but it can make it difficult to swallow when there is inflammation in and around the esophagus. To manage the lubrication, which may be in the form of a sticky, thick, mucus-like phlegm, it is best to stay hydrated. Drinking water, teas or juices constantly will provide your body with adequate fluids which will work to thin out the secretions and make it easier to spit it out if needed.

Constipation

• Drink plenty of fluids unless restricted by your doctor.

• Increase fiber intake to 25-35 grams fiber/day by eating high fiber foods such as Grape Nuts, Shredded Wheat, oatmeal, quinoa, whole grain breads and pastas, beans and lentils.

• Take acacia fiber or psyllium husk powdered supplement. Discuss with your dietitian.

• Get moving! Literally, get up and walk, stretch, be active. This will help move those bowels.

Nurse's Note:
Pain medications can be very constipating. Drink plenty of water and take a stool softener suggested by your physician to help manage this side effect.

• Prunes and dried apricots tend to work well in getting the bowels moving.

• ½ cup prune juice – some like to warm it up.

• Drink fennel tea.

• Consume yogurt daily for the live cultures which will normalize gut flora. May need to take a probiotic supplement daily. First try eating yogurt 1-3 times per day.

Diarrhea

• May try L-glutamine powder. L-glutamine (or just glutamine) is an amino acid that helps repair and heal the lining of the GI tract. Taking 15-30 grams/day for 2 weeks is a decent trial period. Always review use with your dietitian and/or doctor first.

• To replace fluids and electrolytes (sodium and potassium) lost when you have diarrhea, drink water and electrolyte replacement drinks such as Gatorade and Powerade to name a couple of examples. Pedialyte would work also. Be sure to run it by your doctor and nurse to make sure electrolyte drinks are not restricted for any reason.

• Have salty foods such as saltine crackers, broth and pretzels to replace sodium losses.

• Have foods high in potassium such as bananas, tomatoes, carrots, baked potato and plain yogurt to replace potassium losses.

• Increase soluble fiber in your diet such as applesauce, rice, bananas, and oatmeal. Acacia fiber powder is a soluble fiber that works to slowly regulate bowels.

• The only dairy foods you should have when experiencing diarrhea would be yogurt. It is recommended that yogurt be consumed 1-3 times daily to help normalize gut flora. If yogurt is not tolerated, you can take probiotic supplements in the amount of 7-15 billion live cells/day.

• Do not take vitamin C supplements when experiencing diarrhea.

Decreased Or No Appetite

• Try eating small amounts of food more often throughout the day. Make every bite count by choosing high calorie and protein foods such as nuts, seeds, soybeans (edamame), maybe make a trail mix with nuts and dried fruits and even bits of dark chocolate in there. Other suggestions include: hummus spread on carrots, yogurt with low fat granola, whole grain bread with nut butter, hard-boiled egg or cottage cheese and fruit.

• Take Omega-3s daily as they are anti-inflammatory and will help to counteract the inflammatory process that is making you; a) not hungry, and b) when you are hungry you get full fast. Suggest 1500 mg Omega-3 fatty acids (EPA and DHA) daily. Do not take on an empty stomach though. If not able to eat a lot, have a few crackers or half cup of soup before taking supplementation.

• Eat foods high in Omega-3s such as salmon, venison, buffalo, and walnuts, and use flaxseed and canola oils.

• Fruits, especially watermelon, are good to try when you are not feeling very hungry.

• Stay hydrated with water, flavored water, 100% juice popsicles, juices, rice water (congee) and broths.

• Smoothies, shakes and slushies are generally well-tolerated and you can pack in the calories by adding berries, fruits, carrots, milk, yogurt, protein powder, etc.

• You can drink a high calorie nutritional supplement. There are many to choose from and you can even make your own using whey or plant based protein powder. One calorie dense drink I do recommend to gain weight after a big weight loss or to prevent this from happening is Boost (formerly Carnation) VHC (Very High Calorie). This drink, unlike Ensure or regular Boost, is not available retail. You can ask at your cancer care facility or you can possibly contact a local home health company on your own and ask them if they carry this formula or something similar. A solid recommendation is to drink this throughout the day at a ¼ cup dose (equivalent to ¼ can), 4 times per day, refrigerating the formula in between drinks. This will equal one can total per day which is 560 calories. This can help to maintain weight, or at the very least minimize weight loss. What we don't want to happen is significant weight loss. This greatly affects your nutritional status and fighting power.

• An appetite stimulant may be necessary for a brief amount of time. There are a couple we most commonly use, Megace or Marinol. Discuss your appetite with your doctor, nurse and dietitian so that again, we can be proactive in managing your symptoms.

• Try yoga, stretching exercises, deep breathing, Guided Imagery with a licensed counselor, talking with someone or support group, or other means of relieving stress and anxiety that work for you.

Sore Throat/Painful And/Or Difficulty Swallowing

Sometimes radiation may cause some esophagitis. Try

some of these tips to help minimize pain and troubles swallowing.

• Use Magic Mouthwash. It can numb area so that you can swallow.

• Consume mostly soft foods or liquids such as puddings, mashed potatoes, eggs, pasta, oatmeal or other desired hot cereals, protein shakes/smoothies/slushies, canned peaches or pears, yogurts, and cottage cheese.

• Drink milk (skim, soy, almond, or rice milk) between meals. If cancer is estrogenic, 1 cup per day soy milk is allowed.

• Sip soup and teas.

• Make frozen fruit sections (peaches, grapes cut in half, melons) and suck on them.

• There is something called capsaicin taffy. Capsaicin is a pain reliever and it is found in cayenne pepper. You can make it using a small amount of cayenne pepper. NEVER put cayenne pepper directly on your mouth or tongue as it is extremely spicy and hot.

CAPSAICIN TAFFY
1 cup sugar
¾ cup light corn syrup
2/3 cup water
1 tablespoon cornstarch
2 tablespoons soft margarine
1 teaspoon salt
2 teaspoons vanilla
½ to 1½ teaspoons cayenne pepper (powdered)

Begin by using only ½ teaspoon of the cay-enne pepper in the first recipe you make and build up to 1 ½ teaspoons in following batches if it doesn't cause your mouth to burn. COM-BINE: everything except vanilla and cayenne pepper cooking over medium heat stirring constantly, to 256 degrees Fahrenheit (use candy thermometer). Remove from heat and stir in vanilla and cayenne pepper. Once cooled enough to touch, pull taffy. Let cool on wax paper. When stiff, cut into strips, then pieces. Wrap in wax paper and store in cool, dry place.

Dry Mouth/Tender Mouth

• Sip water and teas frequently throughout the day to moisten mouth.

• Limit caffeine and alcohol intake as they tend to be a diuretic and pull fluid out of the body.

• Use a non alcohol containing mouthwash such as Biotene. (big white bottle available at many local retail shops.)

• Have water/water bottle with you at all times—take frequent sips.

• Consume moist foods such as stews, casseroles, soups, and fruits.

• Suck on ice chips, popsicles, or make slushies if cold temperature foods are desired and tolerated.

• Use broth, gravies, sauces, yogurt, silken tofu (moist and creamy), warm water, juices, milk or dairy alterna-

Nurse's Note:

If you use gum, mints, or hard candy to help with dry mouth, choose sugar free as sugar aids in the growth of yeast.

tives, and coconut milk to moisten foods.

• Eat soft foods such as yogurt, all natural ice cream, oatmeal, pudding, Cream Of Wheat, Malt-O-Meal, even cooked vegetables such as cauliflower can be mashed to make "mock mashed potatoes."

• Use olive oil, canola oil, and/or coconut oil to make swallowing easier.

• Avoid crunchy textured foods, tough meats, and raw vegetables.

• Chew xylitol based gum. Xylitol is a sugar-free sweetener and does not promote tooth decay. This is available in most grocery stores down the "health food" or "all natural" sections of the store.

• Use a humidifier in your room at night to keep the air moist.

• Moisten lips frequently with lip balm, Aquafor, cocoa butter or olive oil.

Taste Changes

• Good oral hygiene is a must! Take good care of that mouth. A dry mouth can lead to increased bacteria growth so be sure to keep your mouth moistened and clean. If painful to brush, buy one of those sponge-ended toothbrushes and try using that for brushing.

• Mouthwash can make foods taste better. Rinse well prior to eating and see if this works for you. Biotene as an example of alcohol-free mouthwash that is typically better tolerated than those alcohol-containing mouthwashes.

• For metallic taste and dry mouth try sour food, if tolerated, such as lemon or lime in your drinking water which can work to increase saliva production, too. Eating fruits may also help to get rid of the bad taste.

• Try using plastic ware versus silverware if you have a metallic taste in your mouth.

• Cold foods such as chilled fruit, leaf salads, cold salads (egg, pasta, tuna or quinoa salads) are sometimes better tolerated if you are experiencing bitter or metallic taste changes as well as an "aftertaste."

• Try a variety of teas. Typically hear that mint teas do the trick to lessen bad taste changes.

• Zinc may help minimize or alleviate taste changes. Discuss Zinc supplementation with your oncologist and dietitian.

• Marinate meats, chicken and fish in a sweet marinade —sweet and sour sauce, soy/ginger/honey mixture, or raspberry vinaigrette.

Nausea And Vomiting

• Consume colorless, odorless meals, especially before treatments. Research has shown that the meal you eat prior to treatment can make a difference in how likely you are to experience nausea and vomiting.

• If vomiting, it is most important to focus on keeping adequately hydrated as best you can. Sip fluids every 15 minutes at least. Try clear soda, sports drinks, Pedialyte, juices, popsicles, ice chips, ginger tea or other good-sounding tea, broth, ginger ale. If you are not able to keep things down for 24 – 48 hours, please call your

Nurse's Note:

If vomiting is a problem during treatment, you may need to have IV fluids a few days a week to help support you during this critical time.

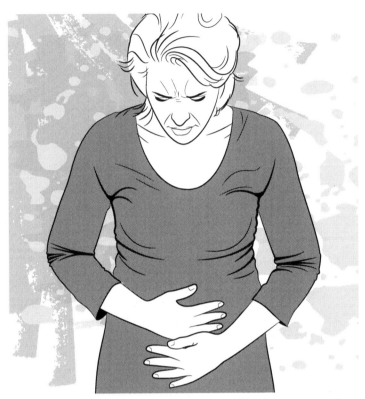

Let your providers know if you are experiencing nausea. With the many new medications available, nausea should not be a big issue for you.

nurse or case manager to let them know.

• Medications are available for nausea management. Discuss these with your oncologist and nurse.

• Eat cold foods as they are generally better tolerated and tend to not trigger vomiting.

• Stick to the old standbys: crackers, dry toast, rice, oatmeal, grits or other hot cereal.

• You can try wearing Sea Bands around your wrist. They hit a trigger point and can help lessen feeling of nausea.

Nurse's Note:

If nausea is an issue, it may help to keep a food diary. This will help you decide which foods to eliminate during therapy to help alleviate side effects.

Anemia

Anemia is when you do not have enough red blood cells. Red blood cells carry oxygen throughout your body and when you do not have enough you may feel tired, weak and/or short of breath. You doctor will be monitoring your lab work to watch for anemia. There are different types of anemia such as iron deficiency anemia or it can be due to low levels of B12 and folic acid. Sometimes anemia is caused by the cancer itself. For iron deficiency anemia, an iron supplement may be ordered by the doctor. It is best to go with a non-constipating iron such as ferrous bis-glycinate. Also try eating high iron foods such as meats, chicken, turkey, or fish. These are called heme sources meaning they come from the blood of the animal. There are non-heme sources like beans, lentils and green leafies. When eating these non-heme sources, have vitamin C with it to increase absorption.

Weight Loss/Gain

During treatment it may become increasingly difficult to manage weight. If having difficulty maintaining weight, continue attempts at eating and drinking as much as possible. As mentioned before, this can be done with sips of water and caloric liquids such as juices, popsicles, smoothies, protein shakes or slushies, etc. If being treated with radiation and/or chemotherapy, esophagitis may occur if it is in the field of radiation making it difficult to eat and drink adequate calories. Do not be alarmed, but a feeding tube may be needed temporarily as a means of nourishing your body until your whole GI tract can be used. It's plain and simple, if you can't swallow your food/liquids you can't meet your nutritional needs. If part of your GI tract is not working properly, nutrition support may be needed. Just know all attempts

Nurse's Note:
Your nurse will weigh you at least weekly during treatment. This may occur more often if weight loss is a concern.

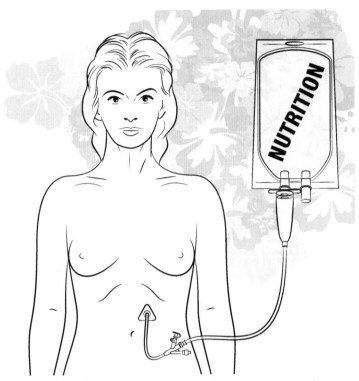

A feeding tube can become a "life-line" for you during radiation treatment if excessive weight loss is a problem.

to help you nourish your body the old fashioned way will be upheld. Be proactive and tell your doctor about any difficulties you may have in maintaining a healthy weight during treatment.

Weight gain is a common complaint made by a breast cancer patient to the dietitian. Weight gain is most likely due to a combination of being thrust into menopause and being less physically active.

Chapter Five

Supplements

The AICR (American Institute of Cancer Research) has made a recommendation to take minimal supplements while increasing nutrient density of your food intake. We do know from recent research that many of us are deficient in vitamin D. Vitamin D deficiencies are linked with cancer, MS, depression, insomnia, aches/pains, etc. Getting your vitamin D tested is highly recommended and from there it can be determined if vitamin D3 supplementation is necessary. A decent maintenance dose is 1000 IU/day, doubling that in the winter months to 2000 IU/day. Testing is necessary to follow up on vitamin D levels to assure there is no toxicity, as well as to be sure adequate amounts of vitamin D3 is taken.

Fish oil, as mentioned, is often recommended because of its anti-inflammatory properties. 1500-3000 mg/day Omega-3s is recommended each day. The Omega-3s are DHA and EPA. Look for the content of these on the back of the supplement bottle. Add up the DHA and EPA to equal the recommended daily dose. Concentrations vary greatly so be sure to take adequate amounts. Carlson brand name offers a quality Omega-3 product. If scheduled to have surgery, be sure to tell your surgeon and all

> **Nurse's Note:**
>
> *Keep a complete list of medications in your wallet or purse. This list should include all natural supplements that you are taking as well.*

physicians involved you are taking fish oil. It is recommended that fish oil be stopped prior to procedures as it thins out the blood.

A multivitamin a day is usually appropriate. Go over contents of it with your registered dietitian and/or doctor. A "clean" product is the best, meaning there are no fillers, preservatives, and maybe even hypoallergenic, using no wheat, soy or derivatives. Some suggestions are Metagenics, Thorne, and Nordic Naturals. These companies offer clean products as do many others. They are only available through a health professional.

A fiber supplement such as acacia fiber, is beneficial if you are prone to constipation or extreme cycles of diarrhea then constipation. If you have increased fiber in your diet by incorporating whole grains, fruits and vegetables, supplementation may not be necessary.

The great debate continues on whether to take antioxidant supplementation during treatment or not. Health care practitioners vary greatly on their stance regarding what is allowed or not allowed during treatment and you will need to discuss this with your oncologist. Listen to your body. You have a mind/body connection and need to listen to it. If you feel confident that something is working for you, do it, as long as treatment is not compromised in any way. Don't do some supplement just because someone told you about it and it worked for them or because of what you read on the internet. You will get tons of advice at every turn, but take time to digest it all and figure out what works for you. Rather than focusing on supplementation for added nutrients, it is better to focus on maximizing your nutrient intake through food.

You can go to www.ORACvalues.com. ORAC stands for oxygen radical absorbance capacity, which is the antioxidant power of foods. *ORACvalues.com* is a comprehensive database of foods and offers a list of determined anti-oxidant levels. Some things high in ORAC are: parsley, blueberries and cinnamon. Check out the website to see what others are high in ORAC values! NOTE: *Always discuss all meds, natural supplements, vitamins and minerals with your doctor to assure nothing is compromising your treatment.*

Recommended Resources

Recommended Books:

Eating Well Through Cancer – distributed by Merck

The Cancer Lifeline Cookbook – by Kimberly Mathai MS, RD, with Ginny Smith

The Cancer-Fighting Kitchen and One Bite at a Time – by Rebecca Katz

In the above-mentioned books you will find whole-foods based recipes and wonderfully helpful nutrition information.

Online Resources:

The world of online information is vast. "Googling" has become a way of life but be careful in what sites you go to. There is one theory found online that gets brought up the most. It is the theory that "sugar feeds cancer."

Please remember one thing: anything growing inside of us will be fueled by what we are fueled by. Our main energy source is glucose. This is sugar. As stated before, follow the 80/20 rule of thumb with regards to diet and nutrition. Most definitely do not avoid fruits and whole grains in hopes of depriving your body of sugar or in hopes of starving the tumor. Keep the focus on balance of carbohydrates, proteins, and good fats. Eat whole grains, bright or dark colored produce, plant proteins, lean or lower fat animal proteins, and good fats.

Recommended Websites:

There are numerous websites to view. So much so it can be overwhelming. Below is a list of credible websites.

www.caring4cancer.com/go/cancer/nutrition - side effects mgmt-written by registered dietitian.

www.cancer.org

www.cancerrd.com

www.cancer.gov

www.nlm.nih.gov/medlineplus

www.aicr.org/site/PageServer

www.mypyramidtracker.gov/planner/

www.oralcancerfoundation.org/dental/xerostomia.htm - information on dry mouth.

www.foodnews.org – for the Dirty Dozen annual report on produce.

www.consumerlabs.com – to review your supplement. See if it passed quality testing.

www.ORACvalues.com – to review antioxidant levels of foods.

www.livestrong.org

www.asha.org/public/speech/disorders/SwallowingProbs.htm - American Speech Language and Hearing Institute.

Journal

Common Cancer Terms

Adenocarcinoma: Cancer that originates from the glandular tissue of the breast.

Adjuvant therapy: Treatment used in addition to the main form of therapy. It usually refers to treatment utilized after surgery. As an example, chemotherapy or radiation may be given after surgery to increase the chance of cure.

Angiogenesis: The process of forming new blood vessels. Some cancer therapies work by blocking angiogenesis, and this blocks nutrients from reaching cancer cells.

Antigen: A substance that triggers an immune response by the body. This immune response involves the body making antibodies.

Benign tumor: An abnormal growth that is not cancer and does not spread to other areas of the body.

Biopsy: The removal of a sample of tissue to detect whether cancer is present.

Brachytherapy: Internal radiation treatment given by placing radioactive seeds or pellets directly in the tumor or next to it.

Cancer: The process of cells growing out of control due to mutations in DNA.

Carcinoma: A malignant tumor (cancer) that starts in the lining layer of organs. The most frequent types are lung, breast, colon, and prostate.

Chemotherapy: Medicine usually given by an IV or in pill form to stop cancer cells from dividing and spreading.

Clinical Trials: Research studies that allow testing of new treatments or drugs and compare the outcomes to standard treatments. Before the new treatment is studied on patients, it is studied in the laboratory. The human studies are called clinical trials.

Computerized Axial Tomography: Otherwise known as a CT scan. This is a picture taken to evaluate the anatomy of the body in three dimensions.

Cytokine: A product of the immune system that may stimulate immunity and cause shrinkage of some cancers.

Deoxyribonucleic Acid: Otherwise known as DNA. The genetic blueprint found in the nucleus of the cell. The DNA holds information on cell growth, division, and function.

Enzyme: A protein that increases the rate of chemical reactions in living cells.

Feeding tube: A flexible tube placed in the stomach through which nutrition can be given.

Gastro Esophageal Reflux Disease (GERD): A condition in which stomach acid moves up into the esophagus and causes a burning sensation.

Genetic Testing: Tests performed to determine whether someone has certain genes which increase cancer risk.

Grade: A measurement of how abnormal a cell looks under a microscope. Cancers with more abnormal appearing cells (higher grade tumors) have the tendency to be faster growing and have a worse prognosis.

Hereditary Cancer Syndrome: Conditions that are associated with cancer development and can occur in family members because of a mutated gene.

Histology: A description of the cancer cells which can distinguish what part of the body the cells originated from.

Immunotherapy: Treatments that promote or support the body's immune system response to a disease such as cancer.

Intensity Modulated Radiation Therapy: Also known as IMRT. A complex type of radiation therapy where many beams are used. It spares surrounding normal tissues and treats the cancer with more precision.

Leukemia: Cancer of the blood or blood-forming organs. People with leukemia often have a noticeable increase in white blood cells (leukocytes).

Localized cancer: Cancer that has not spread to another part of the body.

Lymph nodes: Bean shaped structures that are the "filter" of the body. The fluid that passes through them is called lymph fluid and filters unwanted materials like cancer cells, bacteria, and viruses.

Malignant: A tumor that is cancer.

Metastasis: The spread of cancer cells to other parts of the body such as the lungs or bones.

Monoclonal Antibodies: Antibodies made in the lab to work as homing devices for cancer cells.

Mutation: A change in the DNA of a cell. Cancer is caused by mutations in the cell which lead to abnormal growth and function of the cell.

Neoadjuvant therapy: Systemic and/or radiation treatment given before surgery to shrink a tumor.

Palliative treatment: Treatment that relieves symptoms, such as pain, but is not expected to cure the disease. Its main purpose is to improve the patient's quality of life.

Pathologist: A doctor trained to recognize tumor cells as benign or cancerous.

Positron Emission Tomography: Also known as a PET scan. This test is used to look at cell metabolism to recognize areas in the body where the cancer may be hiding.

Radiation therapy: Invisible high energy beams that can shrink or kill cancer cells.

Recurrence: When cancer comes back after treatment.

Remission: Partial or complete disappearance of the signs and symptoms of cancer. This is not necessarily a cure.

Risk factors: Environmental and genetic factors that increase our chance of getting cancer.

Side effects: Unwanted effects of treatment such as hair loss, burns or rash on the skin, sore throat, etc.

Simulation: Mapping session where radiation is planned. If the doctor will be using a mask for your treatment, this is the time it will be custom fit for your face.

Staging: Tests that help to determine if the cancer has spread to lymph nodes or other organs.

Standard Therapy: The most commonly used and widely accepted form of treatment that has been tested and proven.

Targeted Therapy: Modern cancer treatments that attack the part of cancer cells that make them different from normal cells. Targeted agents tend to have different side effects than conventional chemotherapy drugs.

Tumor: A new growth of tissue which forms a lump on or inside the body that may or may not be cancerous.

About The Authors

Heather Gabbert, MS, RD, LD, CD: Heather attended Southern Illinois University at Carbondale and graduated with her Master's Degree in Dietetics in 1995. She has been a Registered Dietitian (RD) for 17 years and has lived in different areas of the country throughout the years, in each place, gaining valuable experience in the field of dietetics. She has worked with cancer patients since 1998 when she began working at Cancer Treatment Centers of America. She continued to work intermittently for CTCA throughout the many years she has been a practitioner. Heather moved to Spokane, Washington, from Chicago, Illinois, in 2007 where she works as an RD for Cancer Care Northwest and a home health company. Professionally, Heather's passion lies in working with cancer patients and promoting wellness and disease prevention for all.

Heather is a member of Academy of Nutrition and Dietetics (AND), Washington State Academy of Nutrition and Dietetics (WSAND), and Greater Spokane Dietetics Association (GSDA). She served for two years as Media Representative and board member for WSAND and GSDA. Heather has authored a book, been a contributing writer, written articles and was a blogger for StepUpSpokane, highlighting nutrition and wellness. She is a member of AND's DPG groups: Oncology, Business Communications and Entrepreneurs, Dietitians in Integrative Medicine, and Sports, Cardio and Wellness Nutrition (SCAN) group.

Heather most enjoys time spent with her two children. She also enjoys life as a Zumba instructor, exerciser and most memorable activities are her first half marathon and participating in an adventure race, which involved trail-running, biking and kayaking.

Kathy Beach, RN: Kathy graduated with her RN degree in 1993. She decided to get a degree in nursing after her mother was diagnosed with breast cancer. She spent sixteen years in hospital nursing where she worked on a wide range of units from Medical Oncology to Outpatient Surgery. For the past 4 years, she has focused her energy in oncology and radiation oncology with Cancer Care Northwest in Spokane, WA. She loves her work and finds the patients she cares for and their families to be extremely inspiring.

Christopher M. Lee, MD: Dr. Lee is a practicing Radiation Oncologist and is the Director of Research for Cancer Care Northwest and The Gamma Knife of Spokane (Spokane, WA). Dr. Lee graduated cum laude in Biochemistry from Brigham Young University in 1997 which included a summer research fellowship at Harvard University and Brigham and Women's Hospital. He subsequently attended Saint Louis University School of Medicine where he received his M.D. with Distinction in Research degree. He completed four additional years of specialty training in Radiation Oncology at the Huntsman Cancer Hospital and University of Utah Medical Center during which he was given multiple national awards. Dr. Lee has actively pursued both basic science and clinical research throughout his career. He continues to be a proliferative author of scientific papers and regularly gives presentations on radiotherapy technique and the use of targeted radiation in the care of patients with head and neck (throat), brain, breast, gynecologic, and prostate malignancies.

This patient handbook is the breast cancer volume of the "Battling... Cancer with Nutrition" series.

We greatly appreciate the educational grant by:

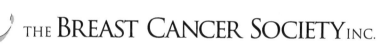 THE BREAST CANCER SOCIETY INC.

which funded the development of this patient-centered guidebook.

Made in the USA
Charleston, SC
05 August 2013